Ketogenic Diet Recipes For Beginners

Introduction

I want to thank you and congratulate you for purchasing the book, *"Ketogenic Diet Recipes For Beginners."*

In order to be successful in adopting any new lifestyle, you need to prepare adequately and the same applies to adopting the ketogenic diet. You want to get all the basics right; have all the ingredients you want as well as all the recipes you can get a hold of. You do not want to find yourself in a situation where you cannot find anything keto friendly to eat.

That is why I wrote this book. This simple guide has 28 tasty ketogenic recipes that you can prepare. In addition, the recipes are simple to make and in a short while, you will have a tasty meal.

Thanks again for purchasing this book. I hope you enjoy it!

The information herein is offered for informational purposes solely, and is universal as so. The presentation of the information is without contract or any type of guarantee assurance.

The trademarks that are used are without any consent, and the publication of the trademark is without permission or backing by the trademark owner. All trademarks and brands within this book are for clarifying purposes only and are the owned by the owners themselves, not affiliated with this document.

Table of Contents

Ketogenic Diet Recipes For Beginners

Introduction

Table of Contents

Breakfast Recipes

Coconut Flour Crepes

Buttery Coconut Flour Waffles

Chocolate Cake Donuts

Strawberry Chocolate Crepes

Egg Crepes with Avocado

Soft Boiled Eggs with Butter and Thyme

Keto Lunches

Baked Pesto Chicken

Shrimp Avocado Salad

Chicken Salad

Crab Stuffed Mushrooms

Tomato Feta Soup

Simple and Tasty Dinner Recipes

Chicken Satay with Peanut Sauce

Coconut-Lime Beef Skirt Steak

Spinach Artichoke Stuffed Chicken Breast

Desserts

Spiced Keto Chocolate

Chocolate Coconut Smoothie Bowl

Pumpkin Cheesecake

Keto Carrot Cake

Orange Cake Balls

Vanilla Pound Cake

Vegan Coconut Macaroons

Almond Joy Chia Seed Pudding

Low Carb Avocado Brownies

Appetizers, Sides, Snacks

Keto Smoothie

Spinach-Mozzarella Stuffed Burgers

Fish Cakes with Avocado Lemon Dipping Sauce

Broccoli Salad

Best Steak Bites Appetizer

Conclusion

Breakfast Recipes

Coconut Flour Crepes

Prep time: 15 minutes

Cook time: 10 minutes

Total time: 25 minutes

Yields: 6 crapes

Ingredients

1 tablespoon of almond meal

2 tablespoons of coconut flour

¼ cup of coconut cream, melted

¼ cup of water or almond milk

1 tablespoon of extra virgin coconut oil, melted

4 eggs

½ teaspoon of vanilla extract

Directions

Add all ingredients to a large mixing bowl in the following order: eggs first followed by the coconut oil, almond milk (or water), coconut cream, vanilla extract, coconut flour and finally the almond meal

Using an electric mixer or whisk, beat the ingredients until you form a smooth batter without lumps. Allow the mixture to sit for 10 minutes so that the coconut flour soaks the liquid to thicken the batter slightly.

Lightly oil a mini egg pan then place over medium/high heat.

Pour ¼ cup of the batter onto the pan. Gently tip and rotate the pan to spread the batter and make it as thin as possible. Brown the bottom side first: cook for 2-3 minutes until it un-sticks easily from the pan and is crispy – the centre should be dry and set before flipping over the crepe to avoid breakage

Cook the other side for about 1-2 minutes and serve hot with your preferred low carb filling such as almond butter, cream cheese, sugar free chocolate chips, sliced almonds, stevia, raspberries etc

*Store leftovers in the fridge on a plate covered with plastic wrap for up to 2 days. Re-warm for a few minutes in the pan before consumption then add filling and enjoy.

Nutritional information per serving: Calories 108, Protein 4.6g, Carbs 2.5g and Fats 8.9g

Buttery Coconut Flour Waffles

Prep time: 10 minutes

Cook time: 20 minutes

Total time: 30 minutes

Yields: 5 waffles

Ingredients

3 tablespoons of full-fat milk

2 teaspoons of vanilla extract

½ cup of melted butter

1 teaspoon of baking powder

4 tablespoons of granulated Stevia

5 eggs (separate the yolks from the egg whites)

4 tablespoons of coconut flour

Directions

Mix the baking powder, Stevia, coconut flour and egg yolks in a bowl

Slowly add the melted butter to the flour mixture and mix well until you get a smooth consistency. Add in the vanilla extract and milk to the mixture. Mix well

Whisk the egg whites in another bowl until fluffy. Gently fold spoonfuls of the whisked egg whites into the flour-butter mixture.

Pour the resulting mixture into your waffle maker and cook until golden brown

Nutritional information per serving: Calories 278, Protein 8g, Carbs 7g and Fat 26g

Chocolate Cake Donuts

Prep time: 15 minutes

Cook time: 18 minutes

Total time: 33 minutes

Yields: 8 servings

Ingredients

Donuts

½ teaspoon of vanilla extract

¼ cup of butter, melted

4 large eggs

¼ teaspoon of salt

1 teaspoon of baking powder

3 tablespoons of cocoa powder

1/3 cup of stevia sweetener

6 tablespoons of water to intensify the chocolate flavor

1/3 cup of coconut flour

Glaze

1 ½ - 2 tablespoons of water

¼ teaspoon of vanilla extract

1 tablespoon of heavy cream

1 tablespoon of cocoa powder

¼ cup of powdered Stevia sweetener

Directions

Donuts

Preheat your oven to 325 degrees F. Grease a donut pan well.

Whisk together the coconut flour, baking powder, salt, cocoa powder and sweetener in a medium bowl. Stir in the vanilla extract, melted butter and eggs then add the cold coffee (or water) and stir until well combined.

Divide the batter equally among the wells of your greased donut pan; you may need to work in batches if you have a six-well donut pan

Bake until the donuts are set and firm to your touch for 16-20 minutes. Remove from the oven and allow the donuts to cool in the rack for 10 minutes before flipping them onto a wire rack to cool completely

Glaze

Whisk together the cocoa powder and powdered sweetener in a medium shallow bowl. Add in the vanilla and heavy cream then whisk to combine.

Add water until the glaze thins out to a "dippable" consistency but is not too watery.

Dip the top of all donuts in the glaze and allow to set – takes about 30 minutes

Nutritional information per serving: Calories 123, Protein 4.43g, Carbs 4.68g and Fats 9.2g

Strawberry Chocolate Crepes

Prep time: 5 minutes

Cook time: 10 minutes

Total time: 15 minutes

Yields: 2 servings

Ingredients

Crepes

1/3 cup of boiling water

1 tablespoon of psyllium husk powder

1 teaspoon of low carb sweetener (this recipe uses Pyure)

3 tablespoons of coconut flour

3 eggs

Filling

½ cup of diced strawberries or raspberries

½ tablespoon of coconut oil or butter

1 ounce of dark chocolate

Directions

Mix the coconut flour, psyllium husk powder, sweetener and eggs in a bowl. Add in the boiling water and mix until incorporated well.

Add 1 tablespoon of oil to a nonstick pan and set the heat to medium. Add in ¼ - ½ of the mixture to the pan once it is hot and cook until the edges start to brown. Flip over and cook until the other side is golden brown; takes around 3-5 minutes per crepe. Repeat with the remaining dough.

If making strawberry chocolate crepe, add butter and chocolate to a microwave safe bowl and microwave until fully melted in 30-second bursts. Ensure you stir between the bursts otherwise the chocolate may burn.

Fill the crepes with a spoonful of chocolate and a handful of berries. Fold the sides of the crepe to close then top with additional chocolate or berries if desired

Nutritional information per serving: Calories 167, Protein 7g, Carbs 10g and Fats 12g

Egg Crepes with Avocado

Prep time: 5 minutes

Cook time: 10 minutes

Total time: 15 minutes

Yields: 1 serving

Ingredients

1/4 avocado thinly sliced

1 handful of alfalfa sprouts

2 eggs

1 teaspoon of mayonnaise

1 teaspoon olive oil

Few slices of turkey cold cuts, shredded

Directions

In a small-medium pan, heat oil over medium heat.

Crack the eggs into the pan once it is hot and spread them around lightly using a spatula so that they are the completely covering the pan and are the same thickness all around.

Cook until crispy then flip over and cook the other side for one more minute then remove from the pan.

Top with the rest of the ingredients in the centre of the egg crepe and tightly roll up

Nutritional information per serving: Calories 268, Protein 12g, Carbs 4g and Fats 22g

Soft Boiled Eggs with Butter and Thyme

Prep time: 10 minutes

Cook time: 6 minutes

Total time: 16 minutes

Yields: 1 serving

Ingredients

1/4 teaspoon of thyme leaves

Himalayan pink salt to taste

Freshly ground black pepper

1 tablespoon of unsalted butter such as Kerrygold's

3 large eggs

Directions

Boil water in a medium saucepan filled halfway through.

Once the water boils use a large spoon to place the eggs in the water gently one at a time. Set your timer to 6 minutes

Meanwhile, in a microwave safe bowl add 1 tablespoon of butter and microwave for about 20 seconds until melted

Remove the saucepan from the stove once the timer goes off and pour out the hot water carefully while ensuring that none of the eggs fall out. Run cold water over the eggs to stop the cooking process

Peel each egg carefully and rinse to do away with any shell fragments then place them gently into the melted butter.

Add in the thyme leaves as well as pepper and salt to taste. Serve immediately.

Nutritional information per serving: Calories 171, Proteins 8.17g, Carbs 3.58g and Fats 13.55g

Keto Lunches

Baked Pesto Chicken

Prep time: 5 minutes

Cook time: 35 minutes

Total time: 40 minutes

Yields: 4 servings

Ingredients

¼ teaspoon of black pepper

½ teaspoon of salt

8 oz. mozzarella cheese, sliced thinly

3 tablespoons of basil pesto

4 chicken breasts (about 1.5 lb) – sliced widthwise in half to make 8 pieces

Directions

Preheat your oven to 350 degrees F.

Prepare your baking dish by spraying with cooking spray then add in the chicken in a single layer at the bottom and sprinkle with pepper and salt. Spread the pesto on the chicken then add the mozzarella on top.

Bake for 35-40 minutes until the cheese is bubbly and golden and the chicken is 160 degrees. If you want, you can broil it for a few minutes at the end to brown the cheese

Nutritional information per serving: Calories 471, Protein 61g, Carbs 2g and Fats 22g

Shrimp Avocado Salad

Prep time: 15 minutes

Cook time: 5 minutes

Total time: 20 minutes

Yields: 2 servings

Ingredients

1/4 teaspoon of black pepper

1/4 teaspoon of salt

1 tablespoon of olive oil

1 tablespoon of lemon juice

2 tablespoons of salted butter, melted

1/3 cup of freshly chopped cilantro or parsley

1/3 cup of crumbled feta cheese

1 tomato diced

1 large avocado diced

8 ounces shrimp peeled, deveined

Directions

Pat dry the shrimp in a bowl, toss the shrimp with the butter until coated well.

Place your pan over medium heat until hot (takes a few minutes). Place the shrimp in a single layer in the pan then sear for a minute until it begins to turn pink around the edges. Turn the shrimp over and cook until it is cooked through – takes less than a minute

Once the shrimp is ready, transfer the pieces to a plate and let it cool as you prepare other ingredients.

Into a large mixing bowl, add the pepper, salt, olive oil, lemon juice, cilantro, feta cheese, diced tomato and diced avocado and toss to mix.

Add the cooked shrimp and mix. Add additional pepper and salt to taste.

Nutritional information per serving: Calories 430, Protein 24g, Carbs 12.5g and Fats 33g

Chicken Salad

Cook Time: 15 minutes

Total Time: 1 hour 30 minutes

Yield: 6 servings

Ingredients

1/4 cup of chopped pecans

2 tablespoons of fresh dill, chopped

1/2 teaspoon of pink Himalayan salt

2 teaspoons of brown mustard

1/2 cup of mayo

3 ribs of celery, diced

1.5 lb of chicken breast

Directions

Preheat your oven to 450 degrees F and prepare your baking sheet by lining with parchment paper.

Bake the chicken breast for about 15 minutes until cooked through.

Remove the cooked chicken from the oven and let it cool. Cut into bite-sized pieces once the chicken is completely cooled.

Add the chicken, salt, brown mustard, mayo and celery to a large bowl. Toss until the ingredients are well combined and the chicken is fully coated.

Cover the bowl with plastic wrap or a lid and refrigerate for about 1-2 hours until chilled. Add the chopped pecans and fresh dill when ready to serve and toss lightly

Serve chilled.

Nutritional information per one cup: Calories 279, Protein 24.8g, Carbs 1.1g and Fat 19.4g

Crab Stuffed Mushrooms

Prep Time 15 minutes

Cook Time 30 minutes

Total time: 45 minutes

Servings 4 servings

Ingredients

1 tablespoon of chopped fresh parsley

2 tablespoons of parmesan cheese, finely grated

20 ounces of baby bella (cremini) mushrooms (20-25 individual mushrooms)

Salt

Filling:

1/4 teaspoon of salt

1/2 teaspoon of black pepper

1/2 teaspoon of paprika

1 teaspoon of dried oregano

5 cloves of garlic, minced

4 ounces of crab meat, finely chopped

4 ounces of cream cheese, softened to room temp

Directions

Preheat your oven to 400 degrees F and prepare your baking sheet by lining with parchment paper.

Separate the mushroom stems from the mushroom caps and discard the stems. Place the mushroom caps on to the earlier prepared baking sheet leaving a 1-inch distance between them; season with salt.

Combine all the filling ingredients in large mixing bowl then stir until well combined without leaving a trace of cream cheese lumps. Stuff the mushroom caps with the filling and sprinkle the top with parmesan cheese evenly

Bake for about 30 minutes until the stuffing is nicely browned on top and the mushrooms are very tender. Top with parsley and serve hot.

Nutritional information per serving: Calories 160, Protein 9g, Carbs 5.5g and Fats 11g

Tomato Feta Soup

Prep time: 5 minutes

Cook time: 25 minutes

Total time: 30 minutes

Yields: 6 servings

Ingredients

2/3 cup of feta cheese — crumbled

1/3 cup of heavy cream

3 cups of water

10 tomatoes, seeded, skinned and chopped — or two 14.5 oz cans of peeled tomatoes

1 tablespoon of tomato paste — optional

1 teaspoon of dried basil

1/2 teaspoon of dried oregano

1 teaspoon of pesto sauce — optional

1/8 teaspoon of black pepper

1/2 teaspoon of salt

2 cloves of garlic

1/4 cup of chopped onion

2 tablespoons of olive oil or butter

Directions

In a large pot, heat olive oil (or butter) in the Dutch oven over medium heat. Add in the chopped onion and cook stirring frequently for 2 minutes. Add in the garlic and cook for 1 more minute. Add the tomatoes, basil, pesto, tomato paste, oregano, pepper, salt and water. Bring to boil then turn down the heat to simmer. Add in the sweetener.

Cook for 20 minutes on medium heat until the tomatoes are cooked and tender. Blend until smooth using an immersion blender. Add the feta cheese and cream cheese. Cook for another minute.

If necessary, add more salt and serve warm.

Nutritional information per serving: Calories 170, Protein 4g, Carbs 10g and Fats 13g

Simple and Tasty Dinner Recipes

Chicken Satay with Peanut Sauce

Prep Time 15 minutes

Cook Time 15 minutes

Total time: 30 minutes

*Marinating Time: 6 hours

Yields: 4 servings

Ingredients

1 scallion thinly sliced

2 boneless skinless chicken breasts (3/4 - 1 pound total)

10 wooden skewers (soaked for about 30 minutes before use)

Marinade:

1/4 teaspoon of cayenne powder

1/2 teaspoon of ground black pepper

1/2 teaspoon of salt

1/2 teaspoon of curry powder

3 cloves of garlic minced

1/2 cup of full-fat coconut milk

Peanut sauce:

1 tablespoon of lime juice

1 tablespoon of soy sauce

1 tablespoon of olive oil

2 tablespoons of sesame oil

3 cloves of garlic, minced

1/4 cup of natural creamy peanut butter

Directions

Marinating the chicken: Mix the marinade ingredients in a large bowl and stir until mixed well.

Cut the chicken into 1-inch chunks then place in the marinade and stir to coat well. Cover and put in the refrigerator for not less than 6 hours.

Cooking the chicken: Thread the chicken chunks onto the wooden skewers ensuring you leave half of each skewer free for holding.

Place on a large baking sheet in a single layer and bake for 10 minutes at 450 degrees F. Flip the skewers over and bake until cooked through for 5 more minutes. Alternatively, you can also grill the chicken skewers

Making peanut sauce: As the chicken is cooking, prepare the sauce by adding all sauce ingredients to a small saucepan over medium low heat.

Stir the ingredients together until smooth for a few minutes. Keep the sauce warm over low heat and stir occasionally.

Serving: Transfer the cooked chicken skewers to a serving plate then brush with peanut sauce. Top with black pepper (if desired) and sliced scallions.

Serve warm.

Nutritional information per serving: Calories 330, Protein 30g, Carbs 5g and Fats 20g

Coconut-Lime Beef Skirt Steak

Prep Time: 10 minutes

Cook Time: 30 minutes

Total Time: 40 minutes

Yields: 4 Servings

Ingredients

2 lbs. of grass-fed skirt steak (can be cut into sections)

3/4 teaspoon of sea salt

1 teaspoon of red pepper flakes (depends on how spicy you like it)

1 teaspoon grated fresh ginger

1 tablespoon of minced garlic

Zest of one lime

2 tablespoons of freshly squeezed lime juice from one lime

1/2 cup of coconut oil, melted

Directions

Combine the salt, red pepper flakes, ginger, garlic, zest, lime juice and coconut oil in a large bowl and mix

Add the steak then rub/ with the marinade. Once you are done, the coconut oil will harden, it's perfectly normal.

Allow the meat to marinate for around 20 minutes at room temperature.

Transfer the steak to a large skillet; cut in half against the grain if it doesn't fit. Scrape the sides of the bowl if there is some marinade stuck on the bowl and add to the pan. Place the skillet over medium high heat to cook the steak.

Sear the steak for 4-5 minutes per side until it is cooked to your desired doneness.

Slice and serve.

Nutritional information for whole recipe: Calories 661, Protein 35g, Carbs 5g and Fats 54g

Spinach Artichoke Stuffed Chicken Breast

Prep time: 15 minutes

Cook time: 15 minutes

Total time: 30 minutes

Yields: 6 servings

Ingredients

¼ teaspoon of pepper, divided

½ teaspoon of salt, divided

¼ cup of frozen spinach drained, and tightly packed

½ cup of artichoke hearts, thinly sliced

½ cup of Mozzarella cheese, shredded

¼ cup of Greek yogurt

4 ounces of cream cheese, softened

2 tablespoons of olive oil

1 ½ lbs. of chicken breasts (6 4-oz. portions)

Directions

Pound the chicken breast into 1-inch thick then cut down each in the middle using a sharp knife ensuring you are careful not to cut all the way through as you are simply making a pocket for the filling. Sprinkle with 1/8 teaspoon of pepper and ¼ teaspoon of salt

Combine 1/8 teaspoon of pepper, ¼ teaspoon of salt, the Greek yogurt, drained spinach, artichoke hearts, mozzarella and cream cheese in a medium sized bowl. Mix thoroughly until well combined

Fill each chicken breast carefully with equal amounts of spinach artichoke filling. Set aside extra filling, if any until the chicken is almost done.

Add the olive oil and stuffed chicken breasts to a large skillet over medium heat then cover. Cook each side for 7-8 minutes or until your meat thermometer reaches 165 degrees when inserted in the chicken

Add the additional filling to the skillet during the last few minutes of cooking to heat it up. Serve with mashed potatoes, mashed cauliflower, regular rice or cauliflower rice

Nutritional information per serving: Calories 288, Proteins 28g, Carbs 2g and Fats 17g

Desserts

Spiced Keto Chocolate

Prep time: 10 minutes

Cook time: 0 minutes

Total time: 10 minutes

Yields: 28 pieces

Ingredients

25 drops of liquid stevia or monk fruit (to taste)

1/4 teaspoon of vanilla extract

50 grams of cacao butter (about 1/4 cup when melted)

1 pinch fine sea salt

1 pinch black pepper

1/8 teaspoon nutmeg

1/4 teaspoon cinnamon

1/2 cup cocoa powder

1/2 teaspoon chili powder

Directions

Whisk together all dry ingredients in a small bowl. Set aside

Pour the cacao butter in a bowl that is microwave-safe and heat in 30 second increments on high until melted, stirring in between. If you prefer, you can also melt in a double boiler.

Stir in the Stevia and vanilla then pour the resulting mixture into the cocoa powder mixture. Stir until smooth.

Pour the mixture into a lightly greased chocolate mold or divide it between 2 lightly greased mini loaf pans

Allow the mixture to set until firm at room temp. Store at room in an airtight container for up to 5 days or freeze for up to 3 months

Nutritional information per serving: Calories 29, Protein 0g, Carbs 1g and Fats 3g

Chocolate Coconut Smoothie Bowl

Prep time: 5 minutes

Cook time: 0 minutes

Total time: 5 minutes

Ingredients

15-20 drops of liquid coconut stevia (or plain stevia to taste)

2 tablespoons of unsweetened raw cacao powder or unsweetened cocoa powder

3/4 cup full-fat canned organic coconut milk (BPA-free)

A Handful of ice (just enough to thicken)

Directions

Put all the ingredients in a blender and blend well.

Pour in a bowl and add optional garnishes.

You can either enjoy immediately, or chill for 30 minutes in the freezer for a thicker consistency.

Nutritional information per serving: Calories 500, Proteins 26g, Carbs 12g and Fats 38g

Pumpkin Cheesecake

Prep time: 15 minutes

Cook time: 0 minutes

Total time: 15 minutes

Yields: 10 servings

Ingredients

3/4 cup of heavy cream

2 tablespoons of Pumpkin Pie Spice, more to taste

2 teaspoons of pure vanilla extract

1/2 cup of confectioners' stevia

1 – 15 ounce can of unsweetened pumpkin puree

12 ounces of cream cheese, softened

Directions

Combine the pumpkin puree and cream cheese in a large mixing bowl. Cream the two ingredients together using a hand mixer until there are no visible clumps and the mixture is creamy and smooth.

Add the heavy cream, pumpkin pie spice, vanilla extract and stevia and mix until the ingredients are well combined

Refrigerate for 1 hour before serving.

Nutritional information per serving: Calories 215, Protein 3g, Carbs 3g and Fats 18g

Keto Carrot Cake

Prep time: 10 minutes

Cook time: 2 minutes

Total time: 12 minutes

Yields: 2 servings

Ingredients

For the cake

1/2 small carrot, finely grated

1/2 teaspoon of vanilla extract

1 large egg, lightly beaten

1 tablespoon of stevia

1/2 teaspoon of baking powder

1 tablespoon of psyllium husk

2 tablespoons of almond flour

1/4 teaspoon of ground ginger

Pinch of salt

1 tablespoon of melted butter

1 teaspoon of cinnamon

1/4 teaspoon of ground cloves (optional)

For the frosting:

1/2 teaspoon of vanilla extract

1/2 tablespoon of stevia

1 tablespoon of whipping cream

1/4 cup of cream cheese, at room temp

Directions

Combine all the cake ingredients in a mug and mix thoroughly until all ingredients are well combined. You can do this in a food processor or blender too. Microwave for 90 seconds on high then remove the cake from the mug and allow it to cool down completely. Slice the cake into 2 layers and put them somewhere cool.

Add the cream cheese, vanilla extract and stevia to a bowl and whip the ingredients using an electric hand mixer until creamy and smooth. Add in the whipping cream and mix for 5 more minutes. Set aside

Scoop one heaped tablespoon of the cream cheese frosting on top of one layer of the cake then place the other layer on it. Scoop another heaped tablespoon of the frosting and place on the top layer of the cake. Spread the remaining frosting using the back of a spoon in any way you prefer.

You can either serve right away or chill first. The colder the cake, the firmer the cream

Nutritional information per serving: Calories 229, Protein 6g, Carbs 20g and Fats 17.3g

Orange Cake Balls

Prep time: 10 minutes

Cook time: 0 minutes

Total time: 10 minutes

Yields: 15 orange balls

Ingredients

1/2 teaspoon of vanilla

35 drops of Sweetleaf vanilla stevia to taste

1/4 cup of orange juice

1/3 cup of coconut flour + more for rolling

2/3 cup of almond butter

Pinch of pink salt

Zest of 2 navel oranges

Directions

Add all ingredients to a mixing bowl and mix well. Adjust if necessary; if too wet, add a sprinkle of coconut flour. Add a drizzle of avocado oil or a splash of orange juice if too dry. Sweeten to taste.

Using a small cookie scoop, make balls. Squeeze the balls smooth and into shape using your palms.

Roll each ball lightly in a small bowl of coconut flour (about 1-2 tablespoons).

Optional: If you want, chill or freeze for 10 minutes to firm up

Nutritional information per serving: Calories 92, Protein 3g, Carbs 4g and Fats 7g

Vanilla Pound Cake

Prep time: 15 minutes

Cook time: 50 minutes

Total time: 1 hour 5 minutes

Yields: 12 servings

Ingredients

4 large eggs

1 cup of sour cream

2 teaspoon of baking powder

1 teaspoon of vanilla extract

1 cup of granular stevia

2 cups of almond flour

2 ounces of cream cheese

1/2 cup of butter

Directions

Preheat your oven to 350 degrees F.

Prepare a 9 inch bundt pan by buttering generously then set aside.

In a large bowl, combine the almond flour with baking powder and set aside.

Cut the butter into small squares then place in another separate bowl. Add in the cream cheese and microwave the cream cheese and butter for 30 seconds. Ensure you do not burn the cheese. Stir until well incorporated.

Add the sour cream, vanilla extract and stevia to the cream cheese and butter mixture. Mix well to combine.

Pour the wet ingredients into the large bowl with baking powder and almond flour. Mix well. Crack in the eggs and stir well.

Pour the batter onto the earlier prepared bundt pan then place in the oven and bake until a toothpick comes out clean when inserted into the cake – takes about 50 minutes

Allow the cake to cool completely for not less than 2 hours, preferably overnight for best results. It may crumble a bit when you remove it too soon.

Nutritional information per serving (65g): Calories 249, Proteins 7.67g, Carbs 5.23g and Fats 20.67g

Vegan Coconut Macaroons

Prep time: 5 minutes

Cook time: 18 minutes

Total time: 23 minutes

Yields: 24 macaroons

Ingredients

1/2 teaspoon of almond extract

1 teaspoon of vanilla extract

1/2 cup of aquafaba

1/2 cup of monk fruit sweetener (or any other sweetener of your choice)

1/2 cup of almond flour

2.5 cups unsweetened shredded coconut, divided

Pinch of salt

For dipping: 1/2 cup of dark chocolate, melted

Directions

Preheat your oven to 350 degrees F and prepare your baking sheet by lining with a silicon mat or parchment paper.

Place 1 cup of the coconut in the oven to toast for 8 to 10 minutes.

Into a large bowl, add all ingredients including the toasted coconuts and stir until well combined.

Scoop in tablespoonfuls and place onto the earlier prepared baking sheet.

Place the baking sheet in the oven and bake for 18-20 minutes.

Melt the vegan dark chocolate. Dip in the bottoms of the cookies once they are cool to touch and place on parchment paper. Place in the fridge for 5-10 minutes to set – they don't need to be refrigerated if you are not dipping in the melted chocolate.

Serve with your desired milk

Nutritional information per serving: Calories 36, Proteins 0.77g, Carbs 3.84g and Fats 1.94g

Almond Joy Chia Seed Pudding

Prep Time: 10 minutes

Cook Time: 1 hour

Total Time: 1 hour 19 minutes

Yields: 4 servings

Ingredients

1/4 cup of sugar-free dark chocolate chips (optional)

2 cups of unsweetened almond milk or coconut milk

1/3 cup of chia seeds

1/2 cup of unsweetened coconut flakes divided

1/4 cup of powered stevia

1/4 cup of unsweetened cocoa powder

2 tablespoons of roasted almonds, crushed

1 teaspoon of pure vanilla extract

Directions

Add the vanilla extract, stevia, cocoa powder, ¼ cup of the coconut flakes and milk into your blender. Blend until all ingredients are well combined.

Pour the blended mixture into a large mixing bowl then add in the chia seeds. Whisk for 1 to 2 minutes vigorously.

Transfer to 4 individual cups or serving bowl and place in the refrigerator for 1-2 hours.

Top with the remaining ¼ cup of coconut flakes, chocolate chips and almonds if desired.

Serve.

Nutritional information per serving (65g): Calories 204, Proteins 5.05g, Carbs 10.21g and Fats 28.65g

Low Carb Avocado Brownies

Prep Time: 10 minutes

Cook Time: 30 minutes

Total Time: 40 minutes

Yields: 12 brownies

Ingredients

1/2 cup of lily's chocolate chips (melted)

2 eggs

3 tablespoons of coconut oil

4 tablespoons of cocoa powder

1/2 teaspoon of vanilla

1 cup mashed avocado

Dry Ingredients

1 teaspoon of stevia powder

60 ml of stevia

1/4 teaspoon of salt

1 teaspoon of baking powder

1/4 teaspoon of baking soda

3/4 cup of blanched almond flour

Directions

Preheat your oven to 350 degrees F.

Combine the dry ingredients together in a separate bowl and mix until well combined.

Peel the avocados then measure or weigh them. Add them to a food processor and process until smooth.

Add the wet ingredients one at a time to the food processor and process for a few seconds until you have added all wet ingredients to the food processor

Now add in the dry ingredients and process until well combined.

Prepare a 30x20cm (12"x8") baking dish by lining with a parchment paper then pour the batter. Place in the oven and bake for around 30 minutes until a toothpick comes out clean when inserted at the centre of the brownies. The top should be soft to your touch.

Remove from the oven and allow to cool completely before slicing it up into 12 pieces.

Nutritional information per serving: Calories 155, Proteins 4.02g, Carbs 9.78g and Fats 14.05g

Appetizers, Sides, Snacks

Keto Smoothie

Prep time: 5 minutes

Cook time: 0 minutes

Total time: 5 minutes

Yields: 2 servings

Ingredients

1 cup of frozen avocado

1/2-1 lemon, peeled

3/4 English cucumber, peeled

1 inch ginger, peeled

1/2 cup of cilantro

1 cup of baby spinach

1 cup of cold water

Directions

Place all ingredients in a high-speed blender and blend until smooth.

Store in the fridge in an airtight container (such as a mason jar) for up to 3 days.

Nutritional information per serving: Calories 148, Proteins 2g, Carbs 13g and Fats 11g

Spinach-Mozzarella Stuffed Burgers

Prep time: 10 minutes

Cook time: 8 minutes

Total time: 18 minutes

Yields: 4 burgers

Ingredients

2 tablespoons of grated parmesan cheese

½ cup of shredded mozzarella cheese (about 4 oz)

2 cups of fresh spinach, firmly packed

¾ teaspoon of ground black pepper

1 teaspoon salt

1½ lbs. of ground chuck

Directions

Combine the ground beef with pepper and salt in a medium bowl.

Scoop about 1/3 cup of the mixture and shape into 8 patties of about ½ inch thick using dampened hands. Put in the refrigerator.

Add the spinach to a saucepan and heat over medium high heat. Cover with a lid and cook until wilted for 2 minutes.

Drain and allow the spinach to cool. Squeeze the spinach with your hands to extract as much liquid as you can.

Transfer the spinach to a cutting board and chop then place in a bowl. Stir in the parmesan and mozzarella cheese.

Mound about ¼ cup of the stuffing into the centre of 4 patties. Cover with the rest of the patties and press the edges together firmly to seal. Cup each patty and round out the edges using your hands

Press on the top to slightly flatten into a single patty. Heat a grill pan or grill to medium high heat – lightly oil the grill grates if using an outdoor grill

Grill the burgers on each side for 5 to 6 minutes. Serve.

Nutritional information per patty: Calories 414, Protein 36g, Carbs 1g and Fats 29g

Fish Cakes with Avocado Lemon Dipping Sauce

Prep time: 5 minutes

Cook time: 10 minutes

Total time: 15 minutes

Yields: 6 servings

Ingredients

1/4 cup of cilantro (leaves and stems)

1 pound of raw white boneless fish (preferably wild caught and local)

Pinch of chili flakes

Pinch of salt

Neutral oil for greasing your hands, for instance avocado oil

1-2 tablespoons of grass-fed ghee or coconut oil for frying

1-2 garlic cloves (optional)

Dipping Sauce:

2 tablespoons of water

1 lemon, juiced

2 ripe avocados

Pinch of salt

Directions

Add the fish, chili, salt, herbs and garlic (if using) into a food processor and blitz until all ingredients are well combined.

Add the ghee or coconut oil to a large frying pan and place over medium high heat. Swirl the pan to coat with the oil.

Oil your hands then roll the mixture into 6 patties. Add the fish cakes to the pan and cook on both sides until cooked through and golden brown.

Meanwhile, prepare the dipping sauce by adding all sauce ingredients to a blender or small food processor and blitz until creamy and smooth. Taste the mixture and add more salt or lemon juice if desired.

Once done cooking, serve the fish cakes warm with dipping sauce.

Nutritional information per serving: Calories 69, Protein 1.1g, Carbs 2.7g and Fats 6.5g

Broccoli Salad

Prep Time: 25 minutes

Cook time: 0 minutes

Total Time 25 minutes

Yields: 8 Servings

Ingredients

For the salad

1/4 cup of roasted salted sunflower seeds

1/3 cup of red onion, diced

1/2 cup of pitted kalamata olives, halved

1/2 cup of sun-dried tomatoes in olive oil, chopped roughly (oil squeezed out)

1/2 cup of artichoke hearts marinated in olive oil, sliced

5 cups of broccoli, cut into small florets

For the dressing

1 teaspoon of sea salt

1 1/2 teaspoons of dried ground thyme

1 1/2 teaspoons of dried ground basil

1 1/2 teaspoons of fresh garlic, minced

1 3/4 teaspoons of dried oregano

4 1/2 teaspoons of monk fruit (or any other granulated sweetener of choice)

Zest and juice of 1 large lemon

2 cups plain, non-fat Greek yogurt

2 tablespoons of oil from the jar of sun-dried tomatoes

Pepper

Directions

Mix all salad ingredients in a large bowl.

Stir together all the dressing ingredients in a medium bowl.

Pour the dressing over the salad and coat well then cover and refrigerate for not less than 2 hours or preferably overnight to allow the broccoli to absorb the dressing and enhance flavor.

Nutritional information per serving: Calories 182, Protein 5.9g, Carbs 14.7g and Fats 12.4g

Best Steak Bites Appetizer

Prep Time: 5 minutes

Cook Time: 2 minutes

Passive Time: 30 minutes

Total Time: 7 minutes

Yields: 4 servings

Ingredients

1/4 teaspoon of black pepper

1 teaspoon of sea salt

1/2 teaspoon of garlic powder

1 tablespoon of balsamic vinegar

3 tablespoons of olive oil

1 lb beef sirloin (cut into 1.5-inch pieces)

Directions

Make the marinade in a medium bowl by rapidly whisking together all ingredients apart from the steak tips until emulsified and uniform

Add the steak pieces to the bowl and coat well with the marinade then cover and marinate for not less than 30 minutes (you can refrigerate in the marinade if you don't plan on making the steak tips right away).

Turn on the stovetop once you are ready to cook. Place a heavy bottom pan over medium high-to-high heat and heat until a drop of water sizzles when added to the pan.

Add a tablespoon of oil once the pan is hot then carefully place in the steak tips in a single layer. Cook for 30 – 60 seconds without disturbing until the bottom is browned. Flip over and cook until the other side is browned for 30 to 60 more seconds.

Nutritional information per serving: Calories 236, Protein 24g, Carbs 1g and Fats 14g

Conclusion

We have come to the end of the book. Thank you for reading and congratulations for reading until the end.

Finally, if you found the book valuable, can you recommend it to others? One way to do that is to post a review on Amazon.

Click here to leave a review for this book on Amazon!

Thank you and good luck!